I0476576

THE
ACID REFLUX
SOLUTION

How to Get Rid of Heartburn, Indigestion
and Acid Reflux…. For Good!

Angie S

ISBN-10: 1514154803
ISBN-13: 978-1514154809

DEDICATION

For those in search of proper procedures needed to get rid
of acid reflux, heartburn, indigestion.

CONTENTS

INTRODUCTION

I want to thank you and congratulate you for purchasing the book, "The Acid Reflux Solution".

This book contains vital information about acid reflux, heartburn, indigestion and the proper procedures needed to get rid of them. If you are one of the many people that suffer from acid reflux, you may be wondering exactly what it will take to get rid of the discomfort. My goal is to lead you in the right direction towards finding that solution.

CHAPTER 1 - WHAT IS ACID REFLUX?

In addition to being very enjoyable, eating is one of the most important activities in someone's life. Humans are able to taste different kinds of food and appreciate these. Moreover, they can use food to gain energy and nutrients that would be delivered into their body. These strengthen the individual and provide him the capacity to fulfill other activities. The consumption of food is possible through the digestive process.

A significant portion of the digestive system consists of one's esophagus and stomach. The esophagus serves as the pathway of food from the mouth to the stomach. Through peristalsis, or the rapid contraction of the esophagus, the food arrives at the stomach to be further broken down. The stomach contains different enzymes and acids to digest the food. These include hydrochloric acid, pepsins, and other enzymes. All of these contribute to helping the body absorb the nutrients. These building blocks are useful in producing energy that is essential in various metabolic processes.

The lower esophageal sphincter (LES) is located between the stomach and esophagus. This circular muscle is responsible for controlling the esophagus once the food enters the stomach. Initially, this muscle remains open as food flows through it. However, once the food has landed in the stomach, the brain sends a signal to this muscle. To prevent any backflow of food, this muscle tightly closes and remains in the said state until new food passes through the esophagus.

There are cases when the LES is weak or may have problems in properly closing. This may act differently and remain open. In effect, the exposed pathway may cause acids from the stomach to move upwards. This moves back into the esophagus. This reaction is then known as acid reflux.

Heartburn

Once the acid begins to rise upwards the esophagus, the individual may experience a burning sensation. Known as heartburn, this feeling is usually located near the back of the individual's throat and his chest area. Because of the delicateness of the esophagus lining, the sensation is sharp and painful. People experiencing heartburn can also feel sick or taste acid at the back of their throats. This can last for several minutes or as long as a few hours. Heartburn can also be worse if the individual bends or lies down.

To clarify, heartburn does not mean that the individual's heart is actually responsible for the reaction. This is named as such because the burning pain is felt near the chest area. Although some people use "heartburn" and "acid reflux" interchangeably, many consider heartburn as one of the symptoms of acid reflux.

Indigestion

While heartburns are already painful, indigestion can also occur simultaneously with these reactions. Also referred to as dyspepsia, indigestion creates a feeling of discomfort after one eats a meal. This may also come with a burning sensation in the upper stomach. Although indigestion and heartburn may seem to be alike, they are different reactions. Many people tend to confuse these two as they are felt after eating food. Usually, certain kinds of food also trigger these reactions. More will be discussed about this in the incoming chapters. For now, it is important to distinguish the two from one another.

Heartburn can be a symptom of acid reflux or indigestion. Moreover, heartburn is a direct effect of acid reflux. On the other hand, various symptoms may cause indigestion. Acid reflux is only one of part of the possible causes. Other factors, such as the individual's emotional health and conditions like gastritis, may also cause indigestion; hence, indigestion is a more complicated condition. While heartburn and indigestion are different, what is clear for both is that acid reflux does play a role in their occurrence.

Why treat these?

Many people disregard the problems of acid reflux, heartburn and indigestion. Because these conditions can occur regularly, people do not see these as major threats to their daily lives. In fact, while 73% of humans have reported suffering from indigestion and heartburn, at least one out of five people will experience symptoms brought by acid refluxes every week. What's more, over 60 million people in the United States will experience heartburn at least once every month.

While some people quickly recover from these reactions, others are unfortunate to actually have these as underlying symptoms of Gastroesophageal reflux disease (GERD). This chronic form of acid reflux is more severe and can significantly affect an individual's life. This can lead to more problems such as ulcers, scarring and bleeding. In other words, it may cause damages to the digestive tract and may eventually cause inefficient digestion or even failure. It is important to pay attention to acid refluxes, indigestions and heartburns to avoid the development of GERD.

As much as possible, treat acid reflux immediately especially if you notice that this happens on a regular basis. In fact, treatment is recommended if the reflux is experienced at least two or three times every week

In getting rid of acid refluxes, the possibility of experiencing heartburns will dramatically decrease. Without acids climbing the esophagus, it is possible to prevent the burning sensation. It also lowers the occurrence of indigestion caused by acid refluxes. Of course, before learning how to treat and prevent these conditions, it is necessary to understand their causes. This will be discussed in the next chapter.

CHAPTER 2 - CAUSES, SYMPTOMS, AND DIAGNOSIS

Anyone can experience acid reflux. Sex, age and ethnicity will not matter. As food primarily triggers the condition, many people have experienced acid reflux at least once in their lives. While indigestion and heartburn can be caused by acid refluxes, it is interesting to know that various reasons trigger the condition itself.

Causes

A common cause of acid reflux is hiatal hernia. This stomach abnormality happens when the LES and the upper part of the stomach move at an area above the diaphragm. The diaphragm is a muscle that is supposed to separate the stomach from the chest. In fact, this also aids in maintaining the acid content within the individual's stomach.

However, hiatal hernia causes muscles of the surrounding stomach area to be very weak. This then causes the stomach to move upwards and through the diaphragm.

As this will be positioned into the chest cavity, the acid can easily move up the esophagus. Unfortunately, the cause of hiatal hernia is unknown. In fact, some people can even be born with this condition. However, studies have shown that overweight people, women, and those older than 50 are of greater risk for hiatal hernia.

Pregnancy can also cause acid reflux. The baby within the womb can exert more pressure to the stomach; thus, causing acids to rise. Hence, women who are at the second and third trimester of pregnancy are more prone to acid reflux.

Aside from these, one's diet and eating habits are major contributors to acid refluxes. Other causes include obesity, smoking and other lifestyle habits.

Symptoms

Usually, the symptoms of acid reflux begin to be visible after having a meal. Heartburn and indigestion are the primary indicators of acid reflux. This is observed through the burning sensation caused by the rising acid content.

Aside from this, chest pain may also take place. However, if chest pain does occur, you must check if the actual cause of it is acid reflux. Because chest pains can be an indicator for a heart attack, one must take this form of pain seriously and immediately consult a doctor.

Other signs also indicate acid reflux. A bitter or sour taste may be present in the mouth. The person may have difficulty talking as their voice has suddenly become hoarse. While pain may be present after the meal, this can become worse when you are at rest. Coughs and nausea may also occur because of these symptoms. In fact, if these become worse, the symptoms may even trigger an asthma attack. Other symptoms include burping, vomiting blood, regurgitation of acids, dysphagia or the feeling of food stuck in the throat and hiccups.

Diagnosis

If you have experienced the symptoms of acid reflux more than two times within a week, consider consulting a doctor. Other indicators for consultation can also involve not getting relief from the usage of medications. Further tests are necessary to confirm the state of the patient and his acid refluxes. Specifically, these are the following procedures that you may need to undergo:

- **Barium swallowing or the esophagram**

  - This is useful in assessing the presence of ulcers or a narrowed esophagus. The patient would swallow a solution and this would display an image on an X-ray.

- **Ph monitoring**
  – This can determine the level of acidity within the esophagus. A device is placed within this area and will stay there for one to two days. After this period, the amount of acids present in the esophagus can be determined.

- **Endoscopy**

  – This can check for existing problems within the stomach or esophagus. A doctor will insert a long, lighted tube down the patient's throat. To make this less painful, the doctor has to spray anesthesia at the back of the patient's throat. A sedative may also be used. While endoscopy is being performed, a biopsy can be done. Tissue samples would be collected. These are to be observed with a microscope to check for abnormalities and infections.

- **Esophageal Manometry**

– This procedure can help in assessing the functionality of the entire esophagus. This procedure also includes observing the LES.

Once the patient has been confirmed to be suffering from acid refluxes, various steps can be performed to help him. These range from direct ways to address the reaction and methods to prevent it from occurring again.

CHAPTER 3 - HOW TO TREAT ACID REFLUX

People do not really know when acid refluxes are bound to happen. Within a few minutes, a delectable dinner can result to a burning sensation in your chest. Since this is painful, you can feel discomfort and may not know how to respond during the actual event of an acid reflux; hence, it is important to keep some tips in mind to be prepared for these occurrences.

Alkalizing Foods

To counter the acidity, it is best to find alkalizing foods. These foods can neutralize the effects of the acids and produce the less harmful salt. For example, you can obtain a spoonful of baking soda once you sense heartburn. Because baking soda is sodium bicarbonate, this would quickly reduce the burning sensation of the heartburn. The basic pH of the baking soda will neutralize these acids.

To prepare this, mix a single teaspoon of baking soda into a glass of water. This should be less than eight ounces. After stirring, the individual should drink the mixture. This process can be repeated several times. However, it is best to drink a maximum of seven and a half teaspoons of baking soda to avoid too much of the said content. Although this can be an effective remedy, using it can produce too much salt. This can cause side effects like nausea. Another alternative is mustard. Specifically, the patient can directly consume it. Almonds are also recommended in case you feel any heartburn or acid reflux coming.

Anti-inflammatory Foods

Anti-inflammatory foods are also recommended. Ginger, Aloe Vera juice, and other soothing foods can help reduce inflammation occurring in the stomach area. As the irritability of the stomach decreases, it reduces the risk of the sudden opening of the LES. Furthermore, it soothes the irritated esophagus w. To prepare the mixture, a half cup of Aloe Vera juice should be mixed with water. The individual can drink this before meals. However, despite the effectiveness of Aloe Vera, one must remember that this is a laxative; hence, it is best to find an Aloe Vera brand that has removed this laxative.

Fight Acid with Acid

Most of the direct remedies to acid reflux focus on the principle of neutralizing the creeping acid. However, it is also possible to consider countering the acid with acid. Acid reflux can actually be caused by having a small amount of acid in the stomach. With insufficient stomach acid, the LES may also receive a signal to loosen and trigger the acid reflux.

If you believe that this is the cause of your acid reflux, you can then choose this option. You will simply need three teaspoons of apple cider vinegar. Mix this with seven ounces of water and the drink it. Before repeating the procedure, you must see if this does lessen the reflux. If not, it is advisable to use another method to respond to the reaction.

If you begin to feel heartburn after eating a meal, chewing gum can also be beneficial. It is interesting to know that this can stimulate saliva production. In effect, this neutralizes the stomach acids. In addition, this causes frequent swallowing and clears the acids present in the esophagus. Although gum is useful, one must avoid mint flavored ones as these can trigger acid refluxes. Choose fruit or cinnamon flavored gum, instead. The person experiencing the heartburn can chew the gum for 30 minutes after eating.

All of these can be initial reactions to stop the acid reflux from worsening. For best results, these tips can also be done before actual meals. In case the acid reflux still occurs, it is advisable to try certain medications to treat the condition.

Angie S

CHAPTER 4 - ACID REFLUX MEDICATION

Although acid reflux is not usually harmful, it can sometimes be painful and occur repetitively. Here is a list of medication; known to help get rid of the heartburn and indigestion sensations:

Antacids

o Antacids are usually composed of three basic salts. These include calcium, aluminum and magnesium with hydroxide or bicarbonate ions. These help in neutralizing stomach acids. In effect, they can react quickly and can provide relief for mild cases of acid reflux that cause heartburn. Antacids can be a liquid that will coat the esophagus lining. This also reduces the acid content of the stomach. Other antacids are also available as chewable tablets or gums.

o While antacids are useful, these are only effective for immediate treatment. Their effects are very short-lived. In fact, these can only last as long as the antacid is present in the said area. In addition, it is important to take note of the amount of antacid intake. Too much of this can cause side effects like constipation. Aside from these limitations, they will not be able to reduce any inflammation caused by the acids. If ever the antacids do not resolve the acid reflux, it is possible that the patient is experiencing more severe conditions; thus, it is advisable for him to consult a doctor.

H-2-receptor blockers

o H-2-receptor blockers aim to decrease the production of stomach acids. This is effective for mild acid refluxes. Furthermore, they are cheap and are ideal for people who experience acid reflux symptoms several times in a month. These blockers can last longer than antacids; thus, providing more relief. However, it is possible for them to take a longer time to react. Nevertheless, these are useful to lower the possibility of heartburn. Usually, they can work within one hour.

o While H-2-receptor blockers are useful, one should be aware of their side effects. Too much of these blockers can cause diarrhea, vomiting, headache and constipation.

Anti-gas medication

- Some patients can also feel bloated or pressure because of heartburn and indigestion. To resolve this, they can take anti-flatulence drugs. These are usually available as tablets and aid in the breaking down of gas bubbles. This makes them easier to eliminate.

Protein Pump Inhibitors (PPIs)

- PPIs can also help in blocking acid production. Furthermore, they are useful in healing the esophageal tissue. In fact, they are powerful drugs that are used for severe cases of acid reflux. However, because of the strength of PPIs, these are usually provided only through prescription. As these are safe, people experiencing severe acid reflux or even GERD are recommended to consider this drug.

Other Medications

Various medicines can help contribute in controlling and preventing acid refluxes. Prokinetics can strengthen the LES and hasten the emptying of the stomach. Foaming agents are also useful to coat the stomach to avoid acid refluxes.

Possibility of Surgery

In extreme cases, however, doctors can recommend surgery if the acid reflux symptoms do not go away. Depending on the severity of the acid reflux, this can be a symptom of GERD. The patients may undergo two types of surgery.

The first involves the placement of a ring around the lower part of the esophagus. This has magnetic titanium beads that are bound together by titanium wires. This device primarily prevents stomach content from moving backwards and returning to the esophagus. While this can prove to be beneficial, people who are allergic to metals should not take this option. In addition, people who decide to undergo this procedure should not undergo MRI tests.

The second procedure is fundoplication. This aims to prevent the recurrence of acid reflux. Specifically, an artificial valve is made with the upper portion of the stomach. This will be wrapped around the LES for strengthening purposes. In addition, this can repair the hiatal hernia condition of a patient. This is usually performed by cutting the chest or abdomen. While this procedure has a high success rate, this is only recommended for extreme cases of acid reflux or GERD.

While all of these medications are useful, one must take note of his situation as he considers what to use. It is important to take note of the severity and frequency of his symptoms If possible, the doctor can also check the patient and see his condition. It is important to know the case of the patient and treat it as soon as possible. This will decrease the chances of patients developing GERD and having to undergo surgery.

To know if there are any complications, the patient can also see other symptoms that occur along with acid reflux. These include anemia, trouble swallowing, and sudden weight loss.

Of course, there are other alternative methods to combat acid reflux. As the medications can eventually pile up, they may become expensive. Experiencing surgery can be very costly too; hence, one way to treat acid reflux is to monitor one's food intake. Since food can trigger these unwanted reactions, knowing what to eat is advisable.

Angie S

CHAPTER 5 – DIETS TO MINIMIZE ACID REFLUX

As the digestive system is the main site that can possibly trigger acid refluxes, it is important to work from this area and find ways to improve its functionality; hence, it's good to monitor food intake and see what food is beneficial or harmful. Furthermore, it is also advisable to practice effective eating habits to minimize acid reflux problems.

Avoid Food that Promotes Acid Reflux

Fatty and fried food is the primary culprit to triggering acid reflux. In fact, these can promote the relaxing of LES; consequently, enabling stomach acid to flow up the esophagus. Such food also delays the emptying of the stomach. All of these reactions can promote acid reflux that lead to heartburn and indigestion.

It is important to avoid foods with high fat content. French fries, onion rings and other fried foods should be eaten sparingly. Fat from bacon, lard and ham should also be avoided. Gravies, salad dressing and cream sauces would also be part of this list. Of course, even sweet desserts and junk food are known to cause acid refluxes. Likewise, butter, cheese and other dairy products can possibly contribute to acid reflux.

Other kinds of food have components that encourage acid reflux to happen. Chocolate contains methylxanthine that can promote the relaxation of the smooth muscles of the LES. Tangy and spicy foods like chili, garlic and onions can also lead to acid reflux.

Some fruits and vegetables, although very nutritious, can be acidic enough to trigger the acid reflux reaction. These include grapefruit, limes, pineapples, oranges, tomatoes and lemons. Aside from solid food, acidic drinks may cause acid refluxes. Examples are coffee, carbonated beverages and tea.

Of course, the reactions of different people to these may vary. While the human stomach can tolerate most of the mentioned food items, it is still best to practice caution especially if you have had past experiences of acid reflux.

Eat Foods that Lessen Acid Reflux

Do not feel overwhelmed with all the foods to avoid. While there are foods that trigger and worsen acid reflux, some foods can also decrease the unwanted reaction. Fortunately, these foods are very delicious and affordable.

Generally, high protein and low fat foods are part of the anti-acid reflux group. As these provide energy and are quickly digested, these can move faster through the digestive tract. In result, it would not cause too much pressure on the stomach. Oatmeal is a good example of food to eat. This is very healthy and can even absorb fat.

This can also aid in weight loss. Also, oatmeal with raisins can further improve the pH level of the stomach fluids. This is possible as the raisins can absorb the acidity present. Chicken, fish and other kinds of meat are also recommended. You can bake or grill these foods; thus, making them among the healthiest food options. It is wise to avoid frying the mentioned foods.

Aside from protein, increasing fiber intake can help and protect the body from acid reflux. These contribute to the efficiency of the digestion process. Green, leafy vegetables are perfect fiber sources. Celery and broccoli are also good choices. Salads can be great ways to enjoy such vegetables. Be sure to take note of the contents of the salad dressing to avoid unwanted acid reflux. Carbohydrate is also useful in alleviating the condition. Rice and couscous are very filling and may cause less or no risk of refluxes.

People who have experienced acid reflux are also recommended to eat certain fruits. Compared to other fruits, these are less acidic and have a pH level close to 7.0. Melons, apples and other similar fruits are examples. However, while these are safer to eat compared to other fruits, some people have reported experiencing acid refluxes because of them.

Yogurt is another ideal choice. Containing probiotics or good bacteria, these foods can aid digestion. It would also provide protection from harmful bacteria; therefore, this also serves well in preventing indigestion.

Improving Eating Habits

Monitoring food intake is not enough. You should also plan how to eat your required meals effectively. This helps in effectively regulating the digestion process and in preventing the stomach from being very full. It is a simple but effective eating habit that can be performed to reduce acid refluxes.

First of all, chewing food is necessary. There is a reason why saliva is present in the mouths of humans. As it contains the initial digestive enzymes, it is important to utilize it to promote an easier digestive process. This can make the job of the stomach easier and faster. Taking time to eat food is recommended. While you would be able to take time to appreciate the taste of whatever you are eating, this also causes a longer time for the food to be broken down by saliva before moving through the esophagus.

Limiting your beverage intake can also help reduce acid reflux. In drinking too much, the liquid can quickly fill your stomach. This provides an avenue for acid reflux to take place. Therefore, as much as possible, one should control his beverage intake. Small sips would be ideal. If possible, drink in between meals as this is better than drinking during meals.

If the stomach is full, more pressure will be present. This can increase the risk of the LES giving way to acid refluxes; medical professionals recommend less food intake. To avoid becoming too hungry or prevent unwanted weight loss, it is best to plan more frequent meals within the day. Instead of three major meals, one can evenly distribute five smaller meals. This can help the stomach to respond more efficiently to the food intake.

Get Some Rest

Another interesting way to improve eating habits is to rest after eating. Gravity plays a role in acid refluxes. If you decide to go to bed right after eating, the way you are positioned on the bed can make it easier for acid reflux to happen. In fact, lying down can cause the food within the stomach to press harder against the LES. It helps to let the body rest after meals. Thirty minutes to three hours would be plenty of time to help the digestive system with the initial entry of the food. Furthermore, it is best to avoid eating foods when bedtime nears.

Through proper discipline and knowledge, it is possible to prevent the effects of acid reflux. However, to maximize these benefits further, it is best to consider methods that can improve your lifestyle. While controlling your food intake is already helpful, there are more ways to create a healthier life without having to worry about acid reflux and its symptoms.

Angie S

CHAPTER 6 – LIFESTYLE CHANGES FOR BETTER RESULTS

While there are treatments that acid reflux patients can use to respond to their condition, these can possibly only provide temporary solutions to the problem; what you must aim for is to create long-term plans that can permanently reduce or eradicate the problem of acid reflux. To do this, the patient must consider various ways to improve his lifestyle. While this can alleviate his acid reflux condition, changing his lifestyle can also serve many other benefits that can prevent other types of conditions.

Stopping Unhealthy Habits

Smoking can contribute to the occurrence of acid reflux. In fact, cigarettes can cause the LES to relax because of their nicotine content. Once the LES relaxes, this will have the tendency to fail to perform its responses efficiently. Other than this effect, smoking can also stimulate the production of stomach acid causing a possibility to worsen the effects of heartburn.

Similar to smoking, alcoholic beverages can assist in the loosening of the sphincter that will control the passage of food through the esophagus. Other than this, alcoholic beverages also contain toxins that are harmful to the body. If too much is consumed, this can bear harmful effects to the chemicals located in your stomach. The beverages may also react with the stomach fluids; thus, causing stronger acid content to backflow.

Avoid Wearing Tight Clothes around the Waist

Even external forces can put an individual at risk to acid refluxes. Tight clothes can squeeze the abdomen of the individual. This then squeezes the stomach. Because of the constricted area, food may be forced to travel against the LES. With this in mind, someone who suffers from constant acid refluxes should consider wearing looser clothing. It is still possible to be fashionable and feel comfortable. Skirts, elastic waistbands and pants would be ideal. If one must wear tight clothing such as suits because of work, it is advisable for him to change into looser clothing when he arrives home.

Exercise and Lose Weight

Maintaining a healthy body is also beneficial in preventing acid refluxes from happening. As obesity can cause great abdominal pressure, the stomach can push its contents up the esophagus. In fact, according to studies, 35 percent of overweight people can experience heartburn. This means that keeping in shape is a major factor in decreasing acid refluxes that can lead to heartburn and indigestion. Through proper dieting and exercise, it is possible to achieve weight loss.

Avoid Stress

Stress can promote behaviors that may trigger heartburns and acid refluxes. Find time to relax and enjoy amidst the pressures of life. You should be able to cope with the challenges that you face. Reducing stress will allow you to observe more positive effects within your body and mental health. This can also help you avoid negative consequences such as excessive weight gain.

There are many ways to decrease stress. In keeping yourself busy and avoid over thinking about problems or other complicated matter. Exercising, watching movies, or playing games are all forms of entertainment that can keep stress levels down. You can talk to your friends, or even shout your worries away. It is not helpful to bottle up your emotions. In doing so, negative hormones can be continually produced to disrupt the normal processes in the body. This then can eventually lead to unwanted conditions such as acid reflux.

Raise the Head Portion of the Bed

To improve the digestion process, you can opt to elevate the headrest of your bed. This will use gravity to assist the downward movement of food through the digestive tract. For best results, firm items such as blocks can be used to raise the head area. Pillows are less effective as these may be too soft and may exaggerate waist bending. Six to eight inches is ideal for elevation.

It is important to do this tip regularly. If there is any improvement seen after several days, you can gradually decrease the angle of the head position. However, you should return this if the acid refluxes begin to increase again.

Given all these considerations, prevention is a major factor that can be used to get rid of acid reflux. In taking proper care of your body, you may avoid the unnecessary discomfort and pain that acid reflux may inflict including indigestion and heartburn.

A FINAL WORD

I want to take this time out to thank you for purchasing this book! The next step is to take action on the advice you've just read about.

Please Leave a Review

Finally, if you enjoyed this book, please take the time to share your thoughts and post a review on Amazon. It'd be greatly appreciated!

That review and feedback will help me improve the content in my books – and make each and every one more relevant and helpful to you.

Thank you again and good luck!

Angie S